Contents

Editor: Norma Pearce
Medical Editor: Dr Tony Smith
Design: Lloyd Fishwick Associates

ISBN: 0 7279 0213 X

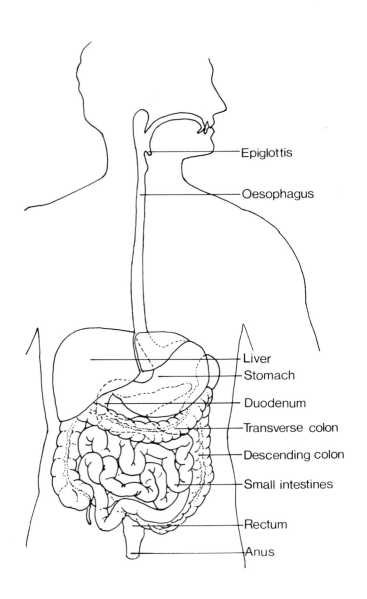

Epiglottis

Oesophagus

Liver

Stomach

Duodenum

Transverse colon

Descending colon

Small intestines

Rectum

Anus

Introduction

Indigestion is an "umbrella" term describing a very common collection of complaints of the stomach and upper part of the digestive system (diagram) that affect most of us at some time and some of us a great deal of the time. The symptoms include pain, heartburn, fullness, regurgitation of food, and wind.

Doctors can often obtain sufficient information to make a diagnosis just by asking you about your symptoms. If, however, your indigestion is sufficiently troublesome to merit a visit to the doctor, and especially if the symptoms persist or recur, you probably need and should have some more detailed investigations to pinpoint the cause and the most effective treatment.

This booklet describes some of the most common causes of indigestion, the investigations that may be carried out, and the treatments available. Indigestion may be caused by:

● **Oesophagitis**—inflammation of the oesophagus or gullet;

● **Gastric or duodenal ulcer**—a small round or oval area which has been worn away in the wall of the stomach (gastric) or the small intestine just below the stomach (duodenum);

● **Cancer of the stomach**—a cancer which, fortunately, is less common now than it was 30 years ago and mainly affects those in late middle age (50–70 years).

● **Non-ulcer dyspepsia (or gastritis)**—indigestion for which no cause can be found, even after full investigation.

Each of these conditions will be discussed in the following chapters, but since lifestyle plays such an important part in the health (or otherwise) of our digestive systems, it is useful to have a look at this first.

Importance of lifestyle

How we live has an important effect on our health. There are a number of abuses to which we subject ourselves and our stomachs that can make us more likely to suffer from indigestion. Equally, however, there are some factors over which we have little control, so if you are troubled by indigestion don't make the problem worse by feeling guilty about having brought it all on yourself!

Diet

The main principles of a healthy diet are to eat less fat and fatty foods, especially those containing animal fats; increase dietary fibre by eating more wholegrain cereals, pulses, and fresh fruit and vegetables; and cut down on sugar and salt.

Food intolerance

Intolerance to certain foods has been considered as one of the causes of non-ulcer dyspepsia (that is, indigestion for which no physical cause can be found). Some people cannot digest foods such as milk or milk products (cheese, yoghurt, etc); others are allergic to certain foods, for example people with coeliac disease, who cannot eat wheat or rye; and some of us may be upset by one constituent of food (for instance caffeine in coffee).

Overweight

Being overweight is considered to be a general health hazard. Oesophagitis, in particular, is often attributed to obesity because this causes flabbiness of the muscles at the lower end of the gullet.

Watch the temperature

Don't eat or drink food or liquid that is too hot as this can cause inflammation of the gullet.

Diet and ulcers

There has been a lot of discussion (without much proof in the way of real facts) about the role of diet in causing ulcers. There have been allegations that diet can both cause and protect against ulcers. It has been shown, for example, that eating too much salt may lead to gastric ulcers and that those who drink a lot of alcohol, coffee, or cola drinks are more likely to develop duodenal ulcers. People who do not eat enough fibre or protein are at higher risk of duodenal ulcers. An increase in the number of people with duodenal ulcers during World War II was attributed to the small amounts of protein available to eat at that time.

Smoking

Smoking aggravates complaints like heartburn because it relaxes the muscles guarding the lower gullet and also slows down the rate at which food is passed from the gullet into the stomach.

Smoking also increases the likelihood of developing both gastric and duodenal ulcers, with the risk depending on the amount smoked. In addition smoking delays the healing of ulcers and increases the chance of them happening again. The risk of dying from an ulcer is six times greater in smokers!

Beware strong drugs!

There is a wide variety of drugs that may damage the lining of the gullet. Injury usually starts within a few days of starting drug treatment. Antibiotics are responsible for over half of the episodes of oesophagitis caused by drugs, but iron pills, vitamin C, aspirin, drugs for arthritis and rheumatism, and many others can cause this disorder.

Oesophagitis caused by drugs can happen at any age and is especially likely if tablets or capsules are washed down with too little fluid or taken just before going to bed. Always take tablets with at least a glass of water and wait for 30 minutes before lying down. If you already have oesophagitis you should take any drugs needed for other illnesses in liquid or soluble form.

Drugs and ulcers

Drugs are also a common cause of ulcers—even a single dose of aspirin, for example, can produce small stomach ulcers in all of us. Other drugs for arthritis and rheumatism are also implicated in ulcer disease. The amount of injury from aspirin and anti-rheumatic drugs is greatest after about one week of continuous treatment. It was shown that approximately 25% of patients attending arthritis clinics who were taking large doses of aspirin had gastric ulcers, but the frequency of ulcers was less with low doses of aspirin and other anti-rheumatic drugs.

Stress

The adverse effects of stress on the digestive system have been shown in a number of excellent studies. Factors such as increased age, male sex, and being unmarried increase the risk of stress and of suffering from abdominal pain. The table, *Life events and stress,* shows the stress levels associated with things such as domestic problems, divorce, bereavement, work problems, and financial difficulties.

Evidence that stress is also harmful for ulcers has been obtained from studies showing that ulcers became a more serious problem during the heavy air raids of World War II and among troops serving in Northern Ireland.

As too much stress has a serious effect on our health and wellbeing it is important to keep it down to manageable levels.

Life events and stress*

Events	Stress rating
Death of spouse Divorce Marital separation Jail term Death of close family member Personal injury or illness Marriage Loss of job	**Highest**
Marital reconciliation Retirement Change in health of family member Pregnancy Sex difficulties Gain of new family member Business readjustment Change of financial state Death of close friend	**High**
Change in number of arguments with spouse Mortgage of over £20 000 Foreclosure of mortgage or loan Change in responsibilities at work Son or daughter leaving home Trouble with in-laws Outstanding personal achievement Wife begins or stops work Begin or end of school Change in living conditions Revision of personal habits Trouble with boss	**Moderate**

*Holmes and Rahe

Oesophagitis

Oesophagitis is the name given to inflammation of the lining of the gullet (oesophagus). The inflammation is usually caused by regurgitation of stomach contents into the lower gullet but sometimes it is a consequence of swallowing drugs prescribed for some other illness (see p 6), or of a hiatal hernia.

How common is oesophagitis?

No-one is quite sure about the frequency of oesophagitis, but a survey of people working in a hospital showed that one in 14 suffered from daily heartburn (a common symptom of the disorder), while one in three complained of at least one attack each month. We have found that about half of the patients attending a hospital clinic for indigestion suffered from oesophagitis, so this is obviously quite a common problem.

Symptoms

Regurgitation of stomach contents (known as *reflux*) is a problem in about two thirds of patients with oesophagitis. Normally the muscles around the lower end of the gullet act as a valve to prevent the contents of the stomach from moving back into the oesophagus, but if these are lax, reflux occurs. Unfortunately reflux itself relaxes these muscles, which weakens the valve action further, and so leads to more reflux—a vicious circle. In addition, the movement of the muscles of the gullet may become abnormal as well as weak, so that food moves into the stomach more slowly than is usual. We do not yet know whether this slowing down is part of the original cause of the oesophagitis or a consequence of the reflux. Finally, the stomach seems to empty too slowly in about half of the patients with reflux, increasing the likelihood that stomach contents will move back into the gullet.

Worse at night

Reflux is usually worse at night and on stooping, especially soon after meals. It can be most unpleasant to wake to find the contents of your stomach on your pillow! You may also have a burning sensation at the back of your throat, hoarseness, or feel as though you have a "lump in the throat", especially first thing in the morning.

Difficulty with swallowing

If you suffer from severe reflux, you may have problems with swallowing food. At first you may have difficulty with solids, and later also with liquids. The food fails to pass into the stomach causing a distressing sensation of "sticking" behind the breastbone. Some patients with swallowing difficulties may have a normal sized gullet, but in others it may be narrowed by scarring.

What aggravates reflux

A number of things seem to make reflux worse. These include eating fat, chocolate, peppermints (which is surprising as many of us eat peppermints to ease indigestion), drinking alcohol, and smoking. Repeated vomiting is also a common cause.

Hiatal hernia

Sometimes reflux may have an obvious physical cause—the condition known as hiatal hernia. Here, however, the symptoms occur both while lying down and when in an upright position.

The hiatus is an opening in the diaphragm through which the gullet passes. If, for any reason, this opening is defective or if the muscles of the diaphragm become flabby or weak, part of the stomach may slip into the

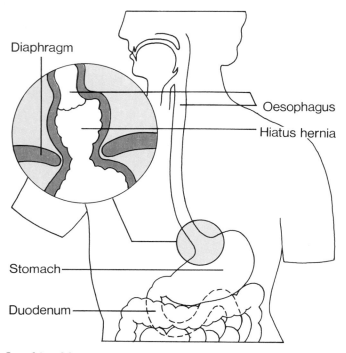

Diaphragm

Oesophagus

Hiatus hernia

Stomach

Duodenum

In a hiatal hernia part of the stomach slips into the chest.

chest. The valve action at the lower end of the gullet cannot then work properly, stomach contents surge into the oesophagus, and it becomes inflamed. This causes further weakening of the muscles surrounding the lower gullet—and another vicious circle.

Nature of reflux

It seems that the type of symptoms suffered depend on the amount of stomach contents regurgitated, how long this is in contact with the lining of the gullet, and on the sensitivity of the lining. Even if the oesophagus is looked at through an endoscope (see p 13) its appearance may not be much of a guide. The lining may look normal in a patient in whom reflux is causing unpleasant symptoms. Conversely, a damaged lining may not give rise to symptoms even when reflux occurs.

Heartburn

Heartburn, as its name suggests, causes an uncomfortable feeling in the region of the heart—the upper abdomen and behind the breastbone. It is a problem in about two thirds of patients suffering from oesophagitis. The discomfort varies in severity and may be made worse by lying down or stooping. Heartburn is often brought on by eating citrus fruits like oranges, lemons, or grapefruit.

Pain

Continuous, periodic, or spasmodic pain in the upper abdomen and behind the breastbone is suffered by about one third of patients with oesophagitis. The pain may be caused or made worse by swallowing.

Bleeding

Occasionally oesophagitis causes sudden bleeding and even the vomiting of blood. Sometimes the bleeding is slight but persistent and in this case the patient may not notice anything is wrong until he or she develops symptoms of anaemia.

Chest complaints

Many patients with oesophagitis wake at night coughing, choking, and spluttering, having inhaled some stomach contents into the lungs. This night-time wheezing is often accompanied by early morning hoarseness and a "lump in the throat", but other complaints usually associated with oesophagitis may be minimal.

Some people with oesophagitis may develop a more serious problem called "gastric asthma", with asthmatic attacks starting at night at times of the year when allergic (related to the amount of pollen in the air) asthma does not occur. There is also an increased likelihood of bronchitis. Patients with gastric asthma benefit greatly from anti-reflux treatment even where reflux is not an obvious problem.

Tests and investigations

If your symptoms suggest that you have oesophagitis the doctor may examine you with an instrument called an endoscope, which allows him to see what is going on inside. A narrow, flexible tube is passed down your throat into the digestive tract. The tube is made up of very skilfully combined glass fibres, down which a powerful light is shone. It is then possible for the doctor to see the whole of the gullet, stomach, and upper small intestine (duodenum). Although this examination may sound pretty grim to you, it is not painful, merely uncomfortable.

Endoscopy often shows reddening and ulceration of the lower gullet in patients with oesophagitis. A biopsy examination of the lining of the lower gullet (taking a very small piece of tissue for examination under a microscope) may detect abnormalities even if the gullet looks normal to the naked eye. Often a hiatal hernia is found during endoscopy in patients with complaints caused by reflux.

Measuring acidity

One of the best tests for oesophagitis involves inserting a small tube with a special tip which can measure changes in the acidity of the contents of the gullet. (As the stomach produces acid, the level of acidity in the gullet will increase if reflux of stomach contents occurs.) The tube is passed through the patient's nose into the gullet where it remains for 24 hours. The acidity measurements are automatically recorded on a small portable recorder the size of a hand-held transistor radio. If you have oesophagitis your gullet will contain more acid and for longer periods of time than is normal. This 24 hour measurement often confirms reflux in patients whose gullet looked normal during endoscopic examination.

Endoscopy

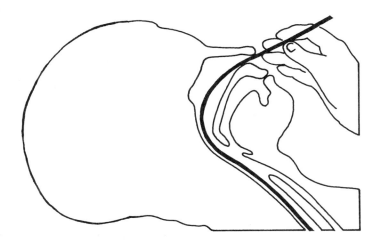

Slow food!

It is also easy for the doctor to measure the rate at which food passes through your gullet. You will be asked to eat some food injected with small amounts of harmless, radioactive material, and the progress of the food through the gullet will be monitored. This investigation can confirm the slowing of the passage of food, and, indeed, food may actually stick and not move at all in some patients whose oesophageal muscle function has been severely damaged by reflux.

Treatment

If you have oesophagitis, you must change your lifestyle if the condition is to improve:

- Eat small meals so as not to overload the stomach;
- Avoid very hot solids and drinks;
- Avoid citrus juices and fruit;
- Don't eat fats and chocolate;
- Cut out alcohol and cigarettes;
- Eat your evening meal early so that your stomach is empty when you go to bed;
- Avoid lying down after meals—allow at least two hours before going to bed;
- It is best not to wear belts or girdles;
- Stooping, especially after a large meal, and heavy lifting are best avoided;
- Lose weight if you are too heavy.

Raise the bedhead

At night it is often helpful to raise the head of the bed by about 20 cm (8 to 9 in) or to use a firm wedge of similar height to raise the chest and head in order to help drain the gullet and lessen the amount of reflux at night. The bed can be raised on wooden blocks or bricks. Increasing the number of pillows does not usually help because you may slide off these during sleep.

Drug treatment

Two types of drug are used to treat oesophagitis—drugs that help to neutralise acids in the gullet (antacids) and those that stop the stomach from producing acid (H_2-antagonists).

Antacids

Antacids are usually the first line of treatment as mild symptoms are often rapidly relieved by these preparations (and they are cheaper than H_2-antagonists). Most doctors prefer to prescribe the type called "raft antacids" (such as Gastrocote, Gaviscon, and Topal) which contain an ingredient that makes the antacid material float to the surface of the stomach contents. When the patient lies down or stoops the antacid raft enters the gullet first and acts as a sort of ball valve.

H_2-antagonists

For more severe oesophagitis you may need drugs that stop the stomach producing acid—H_2-antagonists. These drugs are usually taken after breakfast and also about an hour after an early evening meal (best eaten at about 6–6.30). The drug should be taken in a soluble or dispersable form since tablets may otherwise stay in the gullet for an hour or two, especially if you lie down soon after taking them. It is usually best if the medicines are washed down with a glass of water.

Treatment with H_2-antagonists is only necessary for two or three months in most patients. Recurrences are to be expected, however, especially after late meals or drinks, but these can be treated with a short course of tablets.

Patients who suffer from troublesome heartburn may also need fairly lengthy treatment with H_2-antagonists. Although this continuous treatment may be a nuisance it presents no health risks as H_2-antagonists are remarkably safe.

Drugs that improve muscle tone

If you have severe and persistent symptoms you may get additional benefit from drugs such as Maxolon (metoclopramide hydrochloride) and Motilium (domperidone) that improve the muscles of the oesophagus and stomach. These drugs promote the passage of food down the gullet and also increase the speed with which

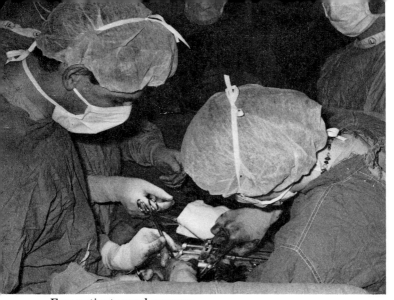

Few patients need surgery.

regurgitated stomach contents leave the gullet and food is emptied from the stomach into the small intestine.

Surgery

A few patients need an operation to reconstruct and tighten the end of the gullet and to repair a hiatal hernia. The risks from this operation are low, complications are uncommon, and the results are satisfactory in at least half of those patients undergoing operation.

Outlook

Inflammation of the lining of the gullet is often difficult to heal completely because the underlying flabbiness of the muscles at the lower end of the gullet cannot easily be corrected. A small proportion of patients develop scarring of the lower gullet and difficulty in swallowing food. This complication is best treated by stretching the narrowed area with an instrument passed through the mouth.

Gastric and duodenal ulcers

Gastric and duodenal ulcers are small, round or oval wounds in the lining of the stomach and duodenum respectively. The duodenum is the first part of the small intestine, just beyond the stomach outlet.

How common are ulcers?

There have been very noticeable changes in the numbers of people suffering from duodenal and gastric ulcers. In many parts of the world, duodenal ulcers have become much less common in men but more frequent in women, perhaps because of the increase in smoking by women. There are still, however, considerable differences in the occurrence of duodenal ulcers within countries. Here, for example, the disease becomes more common the further north you travel— with a very high rate in Scotland.

Unlike duodenal ulcers, gastric ulcers are becoming more common, especially in elderly patients and particularly so in women older than 60. People of this age are more likely to need drug treatment for arthritis and rheumatism, and this treatment is the probable cause of their increased tendency to suffer from gastric ulcers.

Causes

No-one has yet determined exactly why these ulcers occur. The most widely held view is that they are caused by over-production of stomach juices. Gastric juice contains hydrochloric acid and an enzyme, pepsin—a very powerful erosive combination. When the stomach makes too much of these the patient commonly develops one or more ulcers. But if the amounts of acid and pepsin are reduced substantially these ulcers usually heal. Many patients with gastric or duodenal ulcers produce normal amounts of gastric juices, however, so other causes for the ulcers have been sought.

Infections

It has been suggested that factors in our environment may cause ulcers. Among the possible culprits are infectious agents, and recent research has suggested that some bacterial or viral infections may be important. The bacterium *Campylobacter pyloridis* has been implicated, and it has also been proposed that the herpes virus (which causes cold sores) may, in some circumstances, cause duodenal ulcers.

Food and drugs

Some doctors have suggested that eating too much salt may increase the risk of gastric ulcers, and, as we have already seen, aspirin and drugs used to treat arthritis have also been linked with gastric ulcers.

Other factors

Coffee, cola drinks, and emotional stress are powerful stimulants of gastric acid production, although the relevance of this in ulcer disease is not known. Smoking is certainly implicated, particularly in causing relapses.

Symptoms

Pain in the central, upper abdomen, just under the rib margin is the most common complaint and affects nearly all patients. Patients with a gastric ulcer have often suffered from pain for a shorter period (less than one year) than patients with a duodenal ulcer, who have often complained of pain on and off for many years. Other less common symptoms include nausea, vomiting, or heartburn caused by reflux.

The nature of the pain

The pain of ulcers is normally relieved by eating and by antacid preparations, although in some patients, especially those with gastric ulcers, food may actually make it worse. In duodenal ulcers, even if eating helps temporarily, pain often returns 20 to 30 minutes afterwards.

It is often easier to pinpoint the exact site of the pain in duodenal ulcers than in gastric ulcers, and, in addition, the pain of a duodenal ulcer causes waking in the night in two out of three sufferers.

Complications of "silent ulcers"

Sometimes ulcers do not cause pain. These "silent ulcers" are most common in patients who have been taking drugs for arthritis or rheumatism. The ulcers often persist without any problem for some time, but occasionally they may bleed or perforate. Bleeding from an ulcer usually causes vomiting of blood or the passage of black, tarry stools. Perforation means that the ulcer has eaten through the whole thickness of the wall of the stomach or duodenum so that the contents of these organs can leak into the abdomen.

Pointers to a gastric ulcer

Loss of appetite is twice as common in patients with a gastric ulcer as it is in those with a duodenal ulcer, and occurs in approximately two thirds of those with a gastric ulcer. If, therefore, you suffer daily pain, which is brought on by eating and is accompanied by a loss of appetite, the ulcer is more likely to be gastric than duodenal—especially if you are elderly and are taking drugs for arthritis or rheumatism.

But don't jump to conclusions

I must emphasise that these symptoms are not restricted to ulcer disease, and may have some other cause; and, conversely, not all ulcer patients suffer from the typical symptoms listed above.

Tests and investigations

Endoscopy is undoubtedly the best investigation for confirming the diagnosis of gastric or duodenal ulcers because the doctor can actually see where the ulcer is, and its size. A barium x-ray is not nearly as good since this test fails to detect up to one third of ulcers. Where a gastric ulcer is found during endoscopy, it is always necessary to obtain pieces of the lining (a biopsy specimen) for examination under a microscope as ulcers of the stomach may be cancerous.

> ### Barium x-rays
> Barium sulphate is a metallic salt that is visible on x-ray pictures. It is used to show up areas of the digestive tract that need investigation. If you need to have an investigation of the gullet, stomach, or small intestine you may be given barium in the form of a drink and x-rays will then be taken when the barium reaches the relevant part of the digestive tract—10 minutes for the oesophagus, after two to three hours for the small intestine.
>
> Barium x-rays are no longer used as widely as they were before endoscopy became routine as they do not always give reliable results.

Treatment

The treatment of gastric and duodenal ulcers is virtually identical. You must not take aspirin or drugs for rheumatism or arthritis (these are known as non-specific anti-inflammatory drugs—or NSAIDs) unless this treatment is absolutely essential. You should stop smoking since this delays the healing of ulcers and encourages relapse. No special diet is necessary but you should ensure that you eat a well balanced diet with enough roughage in it (see table below).

The fibre-rich foods	Average number of grams of fibre	
	in each portion	in each 100 grams
Breakfast cereals		
Bran-based cereals (42 g)	10.5	25
Wheat flakes and biscuit (42 g)	5	12
Muesli-type, oat and crunchy (70 g)	5	7
Puffed rice and flaked corn cereals (28 g)	2	7
Bread (70 g—2 slices)		
Wholemeal or rye	6	8.5
Brown or malted wheatgrain (eg "Granary")	3.5	5
Rice and spaghetti (56 g dry weight)		
Brown rice	2.5	4.5
Wholemeal pasta	5.5	10
Vegetables (113 g)		
Spinach	7	6
Sweetcorn kernels (99 g)	6	6
Green leafy vegetables eg broccoli and green beans	3	3
Root vegetables eg carrots, parsnips or swede	3	3
Salad and other watery vegetables like lettuce and cucumber	up to 2	up to 2
Potatoes—		
baked with skin (200 g)	4	2
chipped (140 g)	1.5	1
boiled or mashed (113 g)	1	1
Fruit		
Dried fruit (56 g)	9	17
Nuts (50 g)	4.5	9
Fresh fruit—1 piece of large fruit (170 g)	4	2.5
Soft fruit eg strawberries and apricots (113 g)	2	2
Pulses (113 g cooked weight)		
Peas	13.5	12
Baked beans	10	7
Butter beans, kidney beans, lentils	7	6

Drug treatment

When you have an ulcer you are at risk from the twin complications of bleeding and perforation, so priority needs to be given to healing the ulcer. Fortunately, we now have available H_2-antagonists, that act by blocking the production of acid, and dramatically increase the rate of healing as well as the proportion of ulcers which heal. Indeed, eight out of 10 ulcers heal within four weeks of the start of treatment, and most of the remainder heal after another month or two. In addition, the pain is usually relieved within 48 hours of starting treatment.

Management of first occurrences

If this is your first episode of ulcer complaints and you are less than 50 you can be treated differently from older patients or those who have had long-standing and recurrent problems. You may be treated with an H_2-antagonist for two months *without* having the diagnosis confirmed by endoscopy. Treatment is then stopped and perhaps as many as one in five patients with a first episode will have no further problems.

If, however, the pain persists for more than a week after the start of treatment or recurs after treatment has stopped, and in any case if you have had previous episodes of ulcer pain or you are over 50, you must be referred to hospital for further investigations to confirm the diagnosis.

Relapses

Treatment of a relapse is usually simple and effective, which is just as well as most ulcers recur—often two to three times a year for many years and perhaps for life. Most relapses are accompanied by pain and occasionally ulcers bleed or perforate, putting health at considerable risk.

There are two ways of treating relapses. Most commonly each episode of relapse is treated with an H_2-

antagonist for four to eight weeks. Unfortunately, however, this regimen does not prevent further relapses so an alternative approach is to keep the ulcers healed using either surgery or continuous, long term drug treatment.

Surgery

Surgery is no longer used in the treatment of uncomplicated ulcer disease because operations are followed by irreversible complications in quite a number of patients. The most common operations performed in ulcer patients were removal of the affected part of the stomach or duodenum or cutting the vagus nerve supply, which controls stomach emptying and acid production (known as a vagotomy). Today, surgery should only be undertaken in the 5% of patients whose ulcers don't heal with drug treatment and those whose occupation makes reliable, long term treatment impossible (for example, sailors and people working abroad in remote places). Most surgeons will suggest vagotomy rather than gastrectomy and this operation is often combined with pyloroplasty—a simple procedure to widen the exit channel from the stomach to the duodenum.

Long term treatment

Continuous, long term treatment (known as maintenance treatment) with H_2-antagonists is the most satisfactory way of dealing with recurrent ulcers. The drug is taken at night, every night, for many years and perhaps for life. Under these circumstances the H_2-antagonist acts as a blanket on smouldering coals and prevents the flames of ulcer relapse from flickering. If treatment is stopped at any time, even for a few days, the ulcer may recur, so patients shouldn't forget their pills when they go on holiday.

Relapses during maintenance treatment

Maintenance treatment works well for most patients, but in a few, especially heavy smokers, relapses occur during the first year or two after healing and despite continuous treatment. These recurrences are quite different from those suffered by patients who are not on maintenance treatment because there is often no pain and the likelihood of bleeding is very small. These ulcers are easily healed by doubling the dose of pills, and after healing maintenance treatment should be continued at the higher dose.

How long need treatment be continued?

Patients whose ulcers stay healed during the first year of maintenance treatment will usually have no further problems as long as treatment is continued. Unfortunately, however long the treatment, it seems at present that eight in 10 of these patients will have a relapse if treatment is stopped and that maintenance treatment must be continued for many years, perhaps for life. Although it may be a nuisance, maintenance treatment is very safe and side effects are exceptionally rare.

Summary

The current treatment of ulcers is extremely good, but some patients will have to take H_2-antagonists for many years.

Outlook

The outlook for untreated ulcer disease is not yet clear. It has been suggested that the disease burns itself out within 15 to 20 years, but other studies indicate that ulcers may recur throughout the life of the affected patient. Since the introduction of H_2-antagonists in 1975, this outlook has changed and we can now look forward to healing ulcers easily ... and keeping them healed.

Stomach cancer

Cancer is the uncontrolled growth of cells that will, if not stopped, spread locally or to other parts of the body. It seems likely that cancer of the stomach is caused by environmental factors, and the most interesting evidence for this comes from "migrant" studies. For example, cancer of the stomach is very common in Japan. The Japanese who migrate to the USA have almost as much cancer of the stomach as those at home, but subsequent generations show a decided decrease in frequency to levels similar to those found among the white United States population. It seems, therefore, that the cause of cancer of the stomach in Japan is related to the environment early in life. Among the foodstuffs that have been implicated are pickled vegetables and smoked or salted fish or meat. Conversely, a diet containing milk and fresh vegetables is thought to protect against this cancer.

How common is stomach cancer?

Cancers of the stomach have become less common in this country over the past 30 years. It seems that this type of cancer is more frequently encountered among poorer people, among men rather than women, and among those in the age group 50–70 years. Cancer of the stomach is also more common in patients who are heavy drinkers and those already suffering from the blood disorder, pernicious anaemia.

Symptoms

It has been estimated that less than one in a hundred patients who seek advice for indigestion will have cancer of the stomach. A history of recent onset of indigestion in a patient older than 50 years, however, should always arouse suspicion of cancer of the stomach, particularly if the pain or discomfort is continuous (lasting more than 14 days) and is accompanied by nausea, vomiting, and weight loss.

The pain of stomach cancer is often severe and is not related to eating. It may be relieved by antacid preparations at first. Bleeding is not common, but anaemia is quite a frequent complaint.

Tests and investigations

If stomach cancer is suspected further investigations should be done promptly, because the sooner the diagnosis the better the outlook for treatment. Any of the symptoms given above in a patient over 50 require early endoscopic examination to determine whether there is a gastric ulcer and if so to take a biopsy specimen so that a diagnosis of simple ulcer or cancer can be confirmed.

Other tests may include a chest x-ray, blood tests, and if a cancer is found, a liver scan or body scan.

Treatment

Surgery is the only form of treatment that can cure the disease, and if treated sufficiently early, nearly eight in 10 patients survive normally for many years. Unfortunately, however, stomach cancer is often not diagnosed until it is quite far advanced. Radiotherapy (treatment with x-rays) will not effect a cure, but it may be used to control unpleasant symptoms in some patients. Drug therapy (chemotherapy) is only useful in about a quarter of patients.

Outlook

The course of this disease is made worse by extremes of

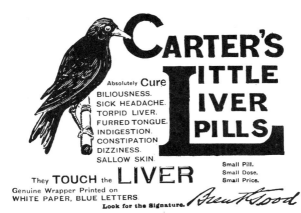
Modern treatments are much more effective than those available to previous generations.

age—being very young or very old; when there is difficulty with swallowing; or if the cancer has spread to other parts of the body.

Gastrectomy

An operation to remove part of the stomach (partial gastrectomy) or all of it (total gastrectomy) may be carried out when the patient has cancer of the stomach.

During the operation you are given a general anaesthetic, and your stomach is sucked clean by a tube passed into your nose and down your oesophagus. The surgeon makes an incision in the upper abdomen and removes part or all of the stomach. The remaining cut edges are then sewn together to maintain a passageway for food.

After the operation you will be fed via a tube, but after a few days your digestive tract should have recovered sufficiently for you to begin eating and drinking again. You will probably be in hospital for 10 to 14 days.

Eating small, frequent meals is often advised after gastrectomy.

Gastritis

Often no cause such as oesophagitis, or ulcers can be found and the terms non-ulcer dyspepsia or gastritis are then used to describe the complaint.

How common is non-ulcer dyspepsia?

Indigestion lasting longer than two weeks is a common cause of disability. One study in the north east of Scotland found that 25% of patients attending their GP suffered from this problem and sickness certificates examined in Sweden showed that "indigestion" was given as the reason in one out of six absences from work.

Symptoms

Approximately 80% of patients suffer from pain in the upper abdomen. The pain often lasts throughout the day and may be a problem at night. Sometimes it is felt in the back. Eating may give relief or make the pain worse. There may be bouts of pain lasting a few weeks or the pain may be continuous for some months.

Many patients with indigestion complain of heartburn, belching, reflux, and a feeling of difficulty with swallowing. Additional problems may be feelings of fullness, upper abdominal swelling, nausea, and intolerance of fatty foods.

Tests and investigations

Patients with indigestion usually have tests for a number of reasons including:

● The necessity of making a firm diagnosis;

- To make sure there is no structural disease;
- To provide a guide for satisfactory treatment;
- To reassure the patient that nothing serious is wrong.

Endoscopy, x-rays, and ultrasound

Patients may be given an endoscopic examination (see p 13), barium meal x-ray examination (p 20), or a trial course of treatment. Endoscopic examination shows that everything looks normal in nearly half of all sufferers, so the doctor can rule out stomach cancer and ulcers. The next step usually is to examine the gall bladder with x-rays or ultrasound (high frequency sound waves that are sent into the body and bounce back showing areas of different densities on a TV screen) to make sure that gall stones are not the cause of the patient's symptoms.

Keeping things moving

Some of us suffer from abnormal movements of the stomach or intestine so that food is not propelled along the intestine in the usual, regular way. Instead there may be "to and fro" movements or simply "laziness" . As there are no really satisfactory tests for these disturbances of movement (or motility), an attempt may be made to relieve complaints by giving a drug that regulates this. If this is a success, it can be assumed that disturbed motility was the cause of the problems.

Treatment

The treatment of indigestion depends on its suspected or confirmed cause. Very often reduction in the intake of alcohol, giving up smoking, or stopping treatment with drugs for arthritis or rheumatism completely relieves the symptoms. Reassurance by the doctor and an explanation of the results of the test helps some patients, as does assistance with any problems that may be causing stress. Occasionally sedative drugs to help combat stress may be beneficial.

Antacids and H₂-antagonists

The treatment of indigestion often depends on the assumption that it is gastric acid that is responsible for the symptoms. For this reason antacid preparations are usually the first line of treatment. In at least a third of patients with indigestion, the symptoms are improved by antacids. In patients whose indigestion is not improved by antacids, H_2-antagonists may be prescribed. These patients should undergo investigations first, however.

The role of campylobacter

The bacterium *Campylobacter pyloridis* has been detected in patients with indigestion and it has been suggested that it plays a part in the problem. As campylobacter is killed by preparations containing bismuth salts these and antibiotics have been prescribed for some patients—successfully in a few.

Drugs for motility

Drugs that regulate the motility of the gullet, stomach, and intestine such as Maxolon (metaclopramide hydrochloride) or Motilium (domperidone) help about one third of patients with indigestion.

Outlook

Indigestion usually continues on and off for many years. Perhaps 10% of sufferers subsequently develop ulcers while about one third are found to be suffering from oesophagitis. It is necessary to carry out the tests all over again if there is any change in the symptoms because the original investigations may have given an inaccurate result (an ulcer may have healed by the time endoscopy was carried out) or some other disease may have developed in the meantime.

About the drugs

I have already mentioned a number of the drugs used in the treatment of ulcers and indigestion. In this section I shall give some more details on the more commonly used drugs because patients like to know what their doctor has prescribed for them and this is not always easy to determine from the name on the packet or bottle.

Antacids

Antacids can often relieve symptoms in non-ulcer dyspepsia and in reflux oesophagitis. They generally contain magnesium or aluminium compounds and act by neutralising the acid produced by the stomach. Antacids should be taken when symptoms occur or are expected—usually between meals and at bedtime, four or more times daily.

It is not possible to list all the antacid preparations that can be prescribed or bought from the chemist without a doctor's prescription. You should experiment until you find one that suits you.

Raft antacids

Raft antacids contain both an antacid and a detergent, and the combination protects against reflux oesophagitis. Some drugs in this category are: Gastrocote (alginic acid) Gaviscon (alginic acid), and Topol (alginic acid).

Motility stimulants

These drugs stimulate gastric emptying and improve the muscle function at the lower end of the gullet. They may be prescribed in reflux oesophagitis and sometimes in non-ulcer dyspepsia where motility problems are considered to be causing the symptoms. Some drugs in this group are: Maxolon (metoclopromide hydrochloride), and Motilium (domperidone).

H₂-antagonists

These drugs heal gastric and duodenal ulcers by reducing the amount of acid produced by the stomach. They are also used in the treatment of oesophagitis and non-ulcer dyspepsia where the patient has been thoroughly investigated and no structural cause for the symptoms has been found. H_2-antagonists are not advised for patients over 50 with undiagnosed indigestion because the drugs may, by reducing symptoms and causing surface healing, delay the diagnosis of a gastric ulcer or perhaps cancer. Drugs in this category are: Axid (nyzatidine), Pepcid PM (famotidine), Tagamet (cimetidine), and Zantac (ranitidine).

Bismuth compounds

Where the bacterium, *Campylobacter pyloridis*, has been found or is suspected as a cause of non-ulcer dyspepsia, a drug called DeNol (tripotassium dicitratobismuthate) may be prescribed.

Conclusions

Indigestion is a common complaint and often there is no obvious cause. Some of the conditions, such as ulcers, which can cause indigestion are a serious, potential threat to health, and so patients with continuous or recurrent symptoms should always undergo full clinical examination and study.